I0436323

"Nature's Pharmacy: Harnessing the Healing Potential of Onions"

Preface

In the intricate tapestry of nature, we often find extraordinary sources of healing concealed within the seemingly mundane. "Nature's Pharmacy: Harnessing the Healing Potential of Onions" unravels the captivating story of a humble kitchen staple that transcends its culinary role to emerge as a potent remedy with remarkable health benefits.

The onion, a ubiquitous vegetable found in kitchens around the world, has been an integral part of human diets for centuries. Yet, beyond its role in enhancing the flavor of our favorite dishes, this unassuming bulb harbors a treasure trove of therapeutic properties. As we delve into the pages of this exploration, we embark on a journey that uncovers the secrets hidden within the layers of the onion, revealing its potential to heal and nourish both body and mind.

This preface sets the stage for a comprehensive exploration of the diverse healing properties found in onions. From traditional remedies passed down through generations to cutting-edge scientific research, "Nature's Pharmacy" illuminates the myriad ways in which onions contribute to our well-being. Through the lens of history, culture, and modern science, we aim to showcase the onion's journey from a culinary staple to a valuable component of holistic health.

As we navigate the pages that follow, readers will encounter a rich tapestry of information, blending ancient wisdom with contemporary insights. The intent is to provide a holistic perspective on the healing potential of onions, touching upon their nutritional value, medicinal applications, and the synergistic relationships between their compounds and the human body.

Ultimately, "Nature's Pharmacy: Harnessing the Healing Potential of Onions" invites readers to rethink the role of this unpretentious vegetable in our lives. It is an invitation to explore the profound connections between nature and medicine, to appreciate the intricate dance of compounds that nature has crafted within the onion, and to consider the ways in which we can integrate this knowledge into our quest for well-being.

Embark on this journey with an open mind and a curiosity for the wonders that nature presents to us. As we uncover the layers of insight within these pages, may we gain a deeper appreciation for the healing potential that lies within the heart of the onion—a treasure waiting to be unearthed in nature's own pharmacy.

Akash Gupta

Chapter 1

Introduction to Alliums: Unveiling Nature's Healing Wonders

In the vast tapestry of nature's offerings, few families of plants captivate both culinary enthusiasts and herbalists quite like Alliums. This diverse family of vegetables, known for its pungent aroma and distinct flavors, includes garlic, leeks, chives, shallots, and the star of our exploration, the humble onion. As we embark on this journey into the world of Alliums, we will unravel the layers of their rich history, nutritional significance, and most notably, their profound contributions to herbal medicine.

The Alluring Allium Family

The Allium family, belonging to the Amaryllidaceae family, encompasses over 700 species, with various members distributed globally. From the delicate chive to the robust garlic bulb, each Allium species brings a unique set of characteristics and flavors to the table. However, it is the onion, scientifically known as Allium cepa, that takes center stage in our exploration of herbal medicine.

Historical Tapestry of Alliums

To understand the significance of Alliums in herbal medicine, we must first journey back through time. Historical records reveal that Alliums have been part of human civilization for thousands of years, cherished for both culinary and medicinal purposes. Ancient Egyptian hieroglyphs and Sanskrit texts from India highlight the use of Alliums in various concoctions, showcasing their esteemed place in ancient herbal traditions.

In ancient Greece and Rome, Alliums were not only prized for their taste but also revered for their purported health benefits. Hippocrates, often hailed as the father of Western medicine, frequently prescribed garlic for its medicinal properties. The Roman naturalist Pliny the Elder documented the use of onions to improve vision and alleviate sleep disorders, contributing to the growing lore of Alliums in the ancient world.

The Medicinal Marvel: Onion

As we narrow our focus to the onion, its medicinal potential becomes increasingly apparent. The onion, with its characteristic layers, serves as a metaphor for the multifaceted benefits it brings to herbal medicine. Rich in sulfur compounds, flavonoids, and essential oils, onions harbor a pharmacological arsenal that modern science continues to unveil.

Sulfur Compounds: Nature's Cleansing Agents

One of the key contributors to the medicinal prowess of onions is their sulfur content. Compounds such as allicin and allyl sulfides are not only responsible for the distinct aroma of onions but also exhibit antibacterial and anti-inflammatory properties. These sulfur compounds play a crucial role in supporting the body's detoxification processes, making onions a natural choice for those seeking to cleanse and revitalize.

Flavonoids: The Antioxidant Guardians

Beyond their pungency, onions boast a rich array of flavonoids, including quercetin, kaempferol, and anthocyanins. These compounds function as potent antioxidants, protecting cells from oxidative stress and inflammation. Research suggests that the antioxidant properties of onions may contribute to cardiovascular health, immune support, and even cancer prevention.

Essential Oils: Aromatherapy for Well-Being

The essential oils found in onions contribute not only to their distinctive scent but also to their therapeutic potential. Thiosulfinates, a class of compounds present in onion essential oils, exhibit antimicrobial properties. Whether inhaled through aromatherapy or consumed, these oils can support respiratory health and provide a natural defense against common pathogens.

Culinary Allure and Medicinal Wisdom

While the medicinal properties of onions are captivating, their culinary allure cannot be overlooked. For centuries, cooks and herbalists alike have harnessed the power of onions to enhance the flavor and nutritional value of dishes. From the delicate sweetness of caramelized onions to the robust kick of raw red onions in salads, the culinary versatility of Alliums is a testament to their enduring popularity.

Navigating the Chapters Ahead

In the chapters that follow, we will embark on a comprehensive exploration of Alliums, with a particular focus on the healing potential of onions. From understanding the biochemistry of onions to exploring their role in traditional medicine practices, each chapter will peel back a layer of knowledge, providing you with insights into the multifaceted benefits of this remarkable herb.

So, as we set forth on this botanical journey, let us embrace the wisdom of the ancients and the discoveries of modern science. Nature's pharmacy awaits, and the onion, with its layers of healing wonders, is our guiding star.

Chapter 2

The Biochemistry of Onions: Unraveling the Molecular Tapestry

As we delve into the world of onion herbal medicine, it's essential to understand the intricate biochemistry that underlies the remarkable healing properties of this humble vegetable. Onions, scientifically known as Allium cepa, are not only culinary delights but also biochemically rich reservoirs of compounds that have been studied for their potential therapeutic benefits. In this chapter, we will peel back the layers of the onion, revealing the fascinating molecules that contribute to its medicinal prowess.

Sulfur Compounds: Guardians of Health

Allicin: Nature's Antibiotic

At the heart of the onion's biochemistry lies allicin, a sulfur-containing compound with potent antibacterial and antifungal properties. When an onion is cut or crushed, the enzyme alliinase converts the precursor compound alliin into allicin. This reaction is a defensive mechanism, as allicin helps protect the onion from pests and pathogens.

In the realm of herbal medicine, allicin is hailed as a natural antibiotic. Studies have shown its efficacy against a range of bacteria, including antibiotic-resistant strains. Its ability to inhibit the growth of harmful microorganisms makes allicin a valuable ally in supporting the body's immune system and promoting overall health.

Allyl Sulfides: Cardiovascular Guardians

Beyond allicin, onions are rich in various allyl sulfides, such as diallyl sulfide, diallyl disulfide, and diallyl trisulfide. These compounds contribute to the characteristic aroma of onions and, more importantly, exhibit cardiovascular benefits.

Research suggests that allyl sulfides may help lower blood pressure, reduce cholesterol levels, and prevent the formation of blood clots. By promoting cardiovascular health, these sulfur compounds play a crucial role in preventing heart diseases and maintaining overall well-being.

Flavonoids: Antioxidant Powerhouses

Quercetin: Nature's Antioxidant

Quercetin, a flavonoid abundantly present in onions, is a powerful antioxidant with anti-inflammatory properties. This compound helps neutralize free radicals in the body, reducing oxidative stress and inflammation. In the context of herbal medicine, quercetin's antioxidant effects contribute to a range of health benefits.

Studies suggest that quercetin may support cardiovascular health by improving blood vessel function and reducing the risk of atherosclerosis. Additionally, its anti-inflammatory properties make it a potential ally in managing conditions such as arthritis and allergies.

Kaempferol: Anti-Cancer Potential

Another noteworthy flavonoid found in onions is kaempferol. Research indicates that kaempferol exhibits anti-cancer properties by interfering with the growth and spread of cancer cells. While more studies are needed to fully understand the extent of its anti-cancer potential, kaempferol adds another layer of complexity to the onion's biochemistry.

Anthocyanins: Colorful Antioxidants

In red and purple onions, the presence of anthocyanins not only contributes to their vibrant hues but also enhances their antioxidant profile. These pigments have been linked to various health benefits, including improved cognitive function and reduced risk of chronic diseases.

Essential Oils: Aromatherapy for Wellness

Thiosulfinates: Antimicrobial Warriors

The essential oils in onions contain thiosulfinates, compounds that exhibit antimicrobial properties. These substances have been shown to inhibit the growth of bacteria, fungi, and even some viruses. In the realm of herbal medicine, thiosulfinates contribute to the onion's role as a natural antimicrobial agent, supporting respiratory health and immune function.

Diallyl Polysulfides: Cellular Protectors

Diallyl polysulfides, another group of compounds derived from essential oils, play a role in cellular protection. These compounds have been studied for their potential in preventing oxidative damage to cells, which is linked to aging and the development of various diseases.

The Synergy of Compounds

What makes the biochemistry of onions truly fascinating is the synergy between these compounds. While each individual component exhibits specific health-promoting properties, their combined effects create a potent cocktail of benefits. The harmonious interplay of sulfur compounds, flavonoids, and essential oils gives onions a multifaceted therapeutic potential that extends far beyond their culinary uses.

Culinary Considerations

Understanding the biochemistry of onions also sheds light on the importance of culinary practices. The way onions are prepared and consumed can influence the bioavailability of these bioactive compounds. For cancer potential, kaempferol adds another layer of complexity to the onion's biochemistry.

Anthocyanins: Colorful Antioxidants

In red and purple onions, the presence of anthocyanins not only contributes to their vibrant hues but also enhances their antioxidant profile. These pigments have been linked to various health benefits, including improved cognitive function and reduced risk of chronic diseases.

Essential Oils: Aromatherapy for Wellness

Thiosulfinates: Antimicrobial Warriors

The essential oils in onions contain thiosulfinates, compounds that exhibit antimicrobial properties. These substances have been shown to inhibit the growth of bacteria, fungi, and even some viruses. In the realm of herbal medicine, thiosulfinates contribute to the onion's role as a natural antimicrobial agent, supporting respiratory health and immune function.

Diallyl Polysulfides: Cellular Protectors

Diallyl polysulfides, another group of compounds derived from essential oils, play a role in cellular protection. These compounds have been studied for their potential in preventing oxidative damage to cells, which is linked to aging and the development of various diseases.

The Synergy of Compounds

What makes the biochemistry of onions truly fascinating is the synergy between these compounds. While each individual component exhibits specific health-promoting properties, their combined effects create a potent cocktail of benefits. The harmonious interplay of sulfur compounds, flavonoids, and essential oils gives onions a multifaceted therapeutic potential that extends far beyond their culinary uses.

Culinary Considerations

Understanding the biochemistry of onions also sheds light on the importance of culinary practices. The way onions are prepared and consumed can influence the bioavailability of these bioactive compounds. For instance, chopping or crushing onions and allowing them to sit before cooking enhances the production of allicin. Similarly, choosing red or purple onions over their white counterparts increases the intake of anthocyanins.

Future Directions in Research

While much has been uncovered about the biochemistry of onions, ongoing research continues to reveal new facets of their molecular makeup and potential applications in herbal medicine. The exploration of onion extracts, isolated compounds, and novel formulations holds promise for the development of innovative therapies and supplements.

In the chapters that follow, we will delve deeper into the practical applications of the biochemistry of onions. From cultivating onions with optimal medicinal properties to preparing herbal remedies, our journey into the world of onion herbal medicine will be guided by a thorough understanding of the molecular tapestry that makes onions a true bioactive treasure.

As we peel back each layer, let us marvel at the complexity of nature's design and the therapeutic potential embedded in the biochemistry of onions.

Chapter 3:

Cultivating Healing - Growing Onions at Home Nurturing Nature's Pharmacy in Your Backyard

As we embark on the journey of exploring onion herbal medicine, it's essential to recognize the profound connection between the cultivation of onions and the therapeutic potential they hold. Cultivating healing at home not only ensures a fresh supply of this versatile herb but also allows individuals to actively participate in their well-being journey. In this chapter, we will delve into the art of growing onions at home, offering insights into the cultivation process, optimal varieties, and the symbiotic relationship between gardener and herb.

The Therapeutic Garden: Planting the Seeds of Well-Being

Selecting the Right Onion Varieties

Before delving into the intricacies of cultivation, it's crucial to choose the right onion varieties for your healing garden. Varieties such as Red Creole, Walla Walla, and Yellow Sweet Spanish are known for their sweet and mild flavors, making them suitable for both culinary and medicinal uses. Additionally, selecting organic, non-GMO seeds ensures a foundation of purity for your healing garden.

Understanding Soil and Sunlight Requirements

Onions thrive in well-drained, fertile soil with a slightly acidic to neutral pH. Choose a sunny location in your garden that receives at least 6-8 hours of sunlight daily. Proper soil preparation, including the addition of organic matter such as compost, sets the stage for robust onion growth.

Sowing the Seeds of Healing

Timing Is Everything

Timing plays a crucial role in the success of onion cultivation. Onions can be grown from seeds, sets (small onion bulbs), or transplants. Depending on your preference and local climate, start seeds indoors 8-10 weeks before the last expected frost or sow them directly in the garden when the soil is workable. For those seeking a head start, sets or transplants can be planted in early spring.

Planting Techniques for Success

When planting onion seeds, sow them thinly in rows, covering them with a light layer of soil. For sets or transplants, ensure proper spacing to allow for bulb development. Mulching around the onion plants helps conserve moisture and suppress weeds. As the onions grow, thin them to the recommended spacing to encourage healthy bulb formation.

Nurturing Growth: Watering and Feeding

The Importance of Adequate Watering

Onions require consistent moisture, especially during the bulb-forming stage. Water deeply when the soil is dry to the touch, but avoid overwatering, as onions are susceptible to rot in waterlogged conditions. Consider using a drip irrigation system to provide a consistent water supply without wetting the foliage excessively.

Feeding for Nutrient-Rich Bulbs

To ensure nutrient-rich bulbs, fertilize onions with a balanced, all-purpose fertilizer during their growth stages. Nitrogen is particularly crucial during the early stages, promoting robust foliage development. As the bulbs form, a fertilizer higher in phosphorus supports bulb expansion and maturation.

Companion Planting for Healthier Onions

Allium Allies: Companion Plants for Onions

Embrace the concept of companion planting to enhance the health and vitality of your onion crop. Planting onions alongside Allium allies such as garlic and chives can deter pests that commonly afflict onions. These Allium plants create a natural barrier against insect invaders, reducing the need for chemical interventions.

Interplanting with Beneficial Herbs and Flowers

Beyond Allium companions, consider interplanting with herbs and flowers known for their beneficial properties. Marigolds, for example, can deter nematodes, while basil may protect against certain pests. This strategic integration not only contributes to the overall well-being of your garden but also adds aesthetic appeal.

Harvesting Healing: Timing and Techniques

Signs of Readiness

Knowing when to harvest your onions is crucial for optimal flavor and medicinal potency. Pay attention to the foliage and bulb development. When the tops begin to yellow and fall over, it's a sign that the onions are nearing maturity. Gently push the soil away to check the bulb size and ensure they have reached the desired diameter.

Proper Harvesting Techniques

Harvest onions on a dry day by gently loosening the soil around the bulbs. Lift them carefully, allowing them to dry in the sun for a day or two. Proper curing involves drying the onions in a well-ventilated area until the outer layers become papery. Once cured, trim the tops and roots, leaving a clean, healthy bulb ready for storage or immediate use.

Storage Wisdom: Preserving the Harvest

Curing for Long-Term Storage

For those looking to enjoy the medicinal benefits of homegrown onions throughout the year, proper storage is key. After harvesting, cure the onions in a warm, dry place with good air circulation. This process allows the outer layers to dry thoroughly, extending the storage life of the bulbs.

Selecting Storage Methods

Storing onions in a cool, dark, and well-ventilated space helps prevent sprouting and decay. Mesh bags or open crates work well, allowing air to circulate around the bulbs. Avoid storing onions near potatoes, as the gases emitted by each can accelerate spoilage.

Practical Applications: From Garden to Remedy

Crafting Homemade Remedies

With a bounty of home grown onions at your disposal, explore the art of crafting homemade remedies. From infusions and teas to poultices and tinctures, the healing potential of your garden can be harnessed for a variety of health needs. Each remedy can be tailored to address specific conditions, offering a personalized approach to well-being.

Embracing the Herbal Lifestyle

Cultivating healing at home extends beyond the act of gardening; it encompasses a holistic lifestyle that values the therapeutic properties of nature. Embrace the herbal lifestyle by incorporating home grown onions into your daily meals, infusing your culinary creations with both flavor and wellness.

Future Growth: Sustainability and Beyond

Sustainable Practices for Continual Healing

As you continue to cultivate healing at home, consider adopting sustainable practices to ensure the longevity of your herbal haven. Composting kitchen scraps, using natural pest control methods, and saving seeds for future plantings contribute to a self-sustaining garden ecosystem.

Exploring New Varieties and Techniques

The world of onion cultivation is vast and continually evolving. Stay curious and explore new onion varieties, cultivation techniques, and companion planting strategies. Experimenting with heirloom varieties or trying your hand at seed saving can add a sense of adventure to your gardening endeavors.

Conclusion: A Garden of Well-Being

In the nurturing embrace of your home garden, the act of growing onions becomes a profound journey of cultivating healing. From selecting the right varieties to harvesting and crafting remedies, each step contributes to a garden of well-being—a sanctuary where the therapeutic potential of nature thrives.

As we turn the pages to the chapters ahead, let the lessons of home cultivation echo, reminding us that true healing begins in the soil and flourishes in the hands of those who tend to nature's pharmacy with care.

Chapter 4

Onion Varieties and Their Medicinal Profiles Navigating the Allium Tapestry

As we delve deeper into the world of onion herbal medicine, it becomes apparent that not all onions are created equal. The vast and diverse family of Alliums offers a palette of onion varieties, each with its unique flavor profile and, intriguingly, distinct medicinal properties. In this chapter, we will navigate the rich tapestry of onion varieties, exploring their diverse characteristics and delving into the nuanced medicinal profiles that make them valuable assets in the realm of herbal wellness.

Yellow Onions: The All-Purpose Warriors

Flavor Profile: Robust and pungent

Medicinal Highlights:

- **Antibacterial Properties:** Yellow onions, with their potent flavor and high allicin content, exhibit strong antibacterial properties. These onions are particularly effective in combatting various bacterial strains, making them a go-to choice for immune support.

- **Anti-Inflammatory Benefits:** The sulfur compounds in yellow onions contribute to their anti-inflammatory effects. This makes them beneficial for individuals dealing with inflammatory conditions, such as arthritis or respiratory issues.

Culinary Versatility: Yellow onions are versatile in the kitchen, adding depth to savory dishes through caramelization or serving as a flavorful base for soups and stews.

Red Onions: The Antioxidant Powerhouses

Flavor Profile: Mild and slightly sweet

Medicinal Highlights:

- **Rich in Quercetin:** Red onions, distinguished by their vibrant hue, are rich in quercetin, a potent antioxidant. Quercetin has been associated with various health benefits, including cardiovascular support and anti-inflammatory effects.

- **Anthocyanin Content:** The red color of these onions is attributed to anthocyanins, which contribute additional antioxidant properties. Anthocyanins have been linked to improved cognitive function and reduced risk of chronic diseases.

Culinary Appeal: Red onions add a burst of color to salads and raw dishes, and their mild flavor makes them a delightful addition to various culinary creations.

White Onions: Mild and Mellow

Flavor Profile: Mild and slightly sweet

Medicinal Highlights:

- **Gentle Flavor for Sensitive Palates:** White onions, with their mild taste, are an excellent choice for individuals with sensitive palates. They offer a subtle onion flavor without the robust pungency found in other varieties.

- **Digestive Wellness:** White onions are often recommended for their digestive benefits. Their mild nature makes them more easily tolerated by individuals with digestive sensitivities.

Culinary Harmony: White onions are prized in dishes where a milder onion flavor is desired, such as in fresh salsas, sandwiches, or light salads.

Sweet Onions: Nature's Candy

Flavor Profile: Exceptionally sweet and mild

Medicinal Highlights:

- **Low Pyruvate Levels:** Sweet onions, like the Vidalia or Walla Walla varieties, are known for their low pyruvate levels, contributing to their sweetness. This makes them a delightful choice for those seeking the benefits of onions without the intense pungency.

- **Anti-Inflammatory Properties:** The natural sweetness of these onions is complemented by anti-inflammatory compounds, offering a gentle yet effective option for individuals with inflammatory conditions.

Culinary Delight: Sweet onions shine in dishes where their natural sweetness can be celebrated, such as in caramelized onion tarts, onion jams, or as a topping for grilled meats.

Shallots: Elegance in Every Bulb

Flavor Profile: Mild and sophisticated, with hints of garlic

Medicinal Highlights:

- **Allicin Content:** Shallots, similar to garlic, contain allicin, a compound known for its antibacterial and immune-boosting properties. Incorporating shallots into your diet can provide a milder alternative to the powerful benefits of garlic.

- **Cardiovascular Support:** The cardiovascular benefits of allicin extend to shallots, making them a heart-healthy choice that adds a touch of elegance to various dishes.

Culinary Sophistication: Shallots are prized for their refined flavor and find a place in gourmet recipes, dressings, and sauces, offering a subtle yet complex taste.

Green Onions (Scallions): Delicate Allium Elegance

Flavor Profile: Mild with a fresh, oniony bite

Medicinal Highlights:

- **Digestive Support:** Green onions are gentle on the digestive system, making them a suitable choice for individuals with sensitive stomachs. They can be a flavorful addition to dishes without overwhelming the palate.

- **Rich in Vitamin K:** These onions are a good source of vitamin K, essential for blood clotting and bone health. Incorporating green onions into your diet contributes to overall wellness.

Culinary Freshness: Green onions are versatile and often used as a garnish or incorporated into salads, providing a burst of freshness and mild onion flavor.

Leeks: The Subtle Allure

Flavor Profile: Mild and slightly sweet, with a subtle onion taste

Medicinal Highlights:

- **Digestive Health:** Leeks are known for their prebiotic properties, promoting the growth of beneficial gut bacteria. This makes them a valuable addition to a diet focused on digestive wellness.
- **Antioxidant Content:** Leeks contain antioxidants, including polyphenols, which contribute to their potential anti-inflammatory and immune-supportive properties.

Culinary Versatility: Leeks are versatile in the kitchen, often used in soups, stews, and casseroles, providing a delicate onion flavor that enhances the overall dish.

Choosing the Right Variety for Your Needs

In selecting onion varieties for your herbal garden, consider the specific health benefits you seek and your culinary preferences. Whether you are drawn to the robustness of yellow onions, the antioxidant power of red onions, the mildness of white onions, the sweetness of Vidalia onions, the sophistication of shallots, or the subtlety of leeks, each variety brings its own unique charm to both the kitchen and the medicine cabinet.

Beyond Culinary and Medicinal Boundaries

As we explore the medicinal profiles of onion varieties, it's important to note that the benefits extend beyond isolated compounds. The synergy of compounds within each onion variety contributes to a holistic approach to well-being. Integrating a variety of onions into your diet allows you to experience a spectrum of flavors and medicinal benefits, promoting overall health and vitality.

Culinary Alchemy: Crafting Healing Meals

Recipes Tailored to Onion Varieties

In the chapters to come, we will delve into the culinary alchemy of crafting healing meals tailored to specific onion varieties. From immunity-boosting soups with yellow onions to antioxidant-rich salads featuring red onions, each recipe will showcase the medicinal prowess of these diverse Alliums.

Balancing Flavors for Wellness

Understanding the flavors and medicinal profiles of onion varieties allows for the creation of balanced and intentional meals. The art of combining these flavors harmoniously not only delights the palate but also nourishes the body, creating a culinary symphony of wellness.

Conclusion: A Garden of Medicinal Diversity

As we navigate the rich tapestry of onion varieties and their medicinal profiles, let us embrace the diversity that nature provides. From the robust to the mild, each onion variety offers a unique contribution to our culinary and medicinal repertoire. In the chapters ahead, we will unlock the full potential of these Allium treasures, exploring recipes and remedies that celebrate the healing journey through the world of onions.

Chapter 5

The Art of Onion Harvesting and Storage Preserving the Bounty: From Garden to Pantry

As we immerse ourselves in the world of onion herbal medicine, the journey doesn't end with cultivation. The art of harvesting and storing onions is a critical chapter in the life cycle of these versatile bulbs, ensuring that the bounty of your garden is preserved for culinary and medicinal use throughout the year. In this chapter, we will unravel the nuances of onion harvesting, explore the signs of readiness, and delve into the meticulous art of storage, allowing you to savor the fruits of your labor long after the growing season.

Signs of Readiness: Timing is Key

Observing Foliage and Bulb Development

The art of onion harvesting begins with keen observation of the signs that indicate the bulbs are ready for harvest. Pay close attention to the foliage; as the tops start to yellow and fall over, it signals that the onion bulbs have completed their growth cycle. The outer layers of the bulb will begin to feel papery, indicating maturity.

Gently Testing Bulb Size

Before plucking an onion from the soil, gently push away the earth to expose the bulb. Assess its size and ensure it has reached the desired diameter. For many onion varieties, this ranges from golf ball to tennis ball size, depending on your preferences and the intended use of the onions.

Timing Variations Based on Variety

Different onion varieties may have slightly different harvesting timelines. Sweet onions, for example, are often harvested earlier when their sweetness is at its peak, while storage onions may be left in the ground longer to develop thicker, more protective outer layers.

Harvesting Techniques: Gentle Hands, Healthy Bulbs

Timing Matters: Choosing the Right Day

Select a dry day for onion harvesting to minimize the risk of rot and facilitate the curing process. The absence of rain ensures that the bulbs are not overly moist, reducing the chance of post-harvest diseases.

Loosening Soil and Lifting with Care

To harvest onions, gently loosen the soil around the bulbs with a hand tool, taking care not to damage the delicate skin. Lift the bulbs by grasping the foliage and gently pulling them from the soil. Avoid yanking or twisting, as this can cause bruising and compromise the quality of the bulbs.

Curing in the Sun

After harvesting, place the onions in a well-ventilated area to cure. This allows the outer layers to dry and the necks to tighten, promoting longer storage life. Avoid exposing the bulbs to direct sunlight, as this can lead to sunscald.

Curing Process: Setting the Stage for Storage Success

Creating an Ideal Curing Environment

The curing process is a crucial step in onion harvesting, setting the stage for successful storage. Arrange the harvested onions in a single layer, ensuring good air circulation. A shaded, dry location with good ventilation, such as a covered porch or well-ventilated garage, is ideal for curing.

Patience Pays Off

Allow the onions to cure for a minimum of two weeks, though some varieties may benefit from a more extended curing period. Patience is key during this phase, as the slow drying process contributes to the development of protective layers that enhance storage longevity.

Selecting and Preparing for Storage

Discarding Damaged or Infected Bulbs

Before storing, carefully inspect each onion. Discard any bulbs that show signs of damage, disease, or pest infestation. Removing compromised onions prevents the spread of issues to the entire storage batch.

Trimming Tops and Roots

Trim the tops and roots of the cured onions, leaving about an inch of each. This creates a neat, clean appearance and minimizes the risk of rot during storage. However, leave the protective dry outer layers intact.

Storage Methods: Preserving Freshness and Flavor

Choosing the Right Containers

Selecting suitable storage containers is crucial to preserving the freshness and flavor of your onions. Mesh bags, wooden crates, or well-ventilated baskets work well, allowing air circulation to prevent moisture buildup.

Ideal Storage Conditions

Onions thrive in cool, dark, and dry conditions. Aim for a storage area with temperatures between 32°F and 40°F (0°C to 4°C). Avoid storing onions near potatoes, as both release gases that can accelerate spoilage.

Sorting for Longevity

Sort onions based on size and condition to maximize storage longevity. Use larger, fully mature bulbs first, as they tend to have a shorter shelf life than smaller onions. Plan your meals and recipes to ensure a steady rotation of stored onions.

Practical Applications: Crafting from Your Storage

Incorporating Home grown Onions Year-Round

The art of onion harvesting and storage culminates in the joy of incorporating home grown onions into your meals year-round. From hearty stews in the winter to fresh salads in the summer, your stored onions provide a continuous source of flavor and nutritional benefits.

Crafting Homemade Remedies

Beyond culinary applications, your stored onions become a valuable resource for crafting homemade remedies. Whether preparing onion-infused oils, tinctures, or poultices, the medicinal properties of your homegrown bulbs can be harnessed for various health needs.

Future Harvests: Seed Saving and Sustainability

Saving Seeds for the Next Generation

As you revel in the success of your onion harvest, consider the practice of seed saving for future plantings. Allowing some of your onions to bolt and produce seeds not only contributes to the sustainability of your garden but also ensures a continuous cycle of growth and abundance.

Sustainable Practices for Ongoing Success

Incorporate sustainable practices into your onion cultivation and harvesting routine. Composting discarded foliage and kitchen scraps, using natural pest control methods, and rotating crops contribute to the health of your garden ecosystem.

Conclusion: A Harvest of Wisdom

The art of onion harvesting and storage is more than a practical skill; it's a testament to the wisdom of working in harmony with nature's cycles. As you lift each onion from the soil, cure it with patience, and store it with care, you become a steward of the land, preserving the bounty for the seasons to come.

In the chapters ahead, we will explore the culinary and medicinal applications of your stored onions, unlocking the full spectrum of flavors and benefits that emerge from the artful combination of nature's gifts and the hands that tend to them.

Chapter 6

The Healing Kitchen - Incorporating Onions into Daily Meals From Garden to Table: A Symphony of Flavor and Wellness

As we continue our journey into the world of onion herbal medicine, the kitchen becomes our canvas for crafting meals that not only delight the palate but also nourish the body. In this chapter, we will explore the art of incorporating onions into daily meals, unlocking the full spectrum of flavors and medicinal benefits that these versatile bulbs offer. From savory stews to vibrant salads, the healing kitchen becomes a sanctuary where the therapeutic properties of onions seamlessly merge with the joy of culinary creativity.

Yellow Onions: Robust Foundations for Flavorful Creations

1. **Immune-Boosting Soups:** Yellow onions, with their robust flavor and immune-boosting properties,

form the perfect foundation for hearty soups. Whether crafting a classic French onion soup or a comforting chicken broth, the aromatic depth of yellow onions adds a layer of complexity to your bowl of wellness.

2. **Caramelized Delights:** Transform yellow onions into golden strands of sweetness through the alchemical process of caramelization. Use caramelized onions as a topping for pizzas, sandwiches, or savory tarts. Their rich, sweet flavor elevates the simplest dishes into culinary masterpieces.

Red Onions: Antioxidant Elegance in Every Bite

1. **Vibrant Salads:** The antioxidant power of red onions makes them a colorful addition to fresh salads. Slice them thinly and toss them into a Mediterranean chickpea salad, where their mild sweetness complements the vibrant flavors of cherry tomatoes, cucumbers, and feta.

2. **Pickled Perfection:** Preserve the crisp texture and striking color of red onions by pickling them. These tangy, pickled gems can be served as a condiment alongside grilled meats, added to tacos, or used to brighten up a plate of avocado toast.

White Onions: Gentle Elegance for Delicate Palates

1. **Fresh Salsas:** White onions, with their mild and slightly sweet taste, are ideal for crafting fresh salsas. Combine finely diced white onions with tomatoes, cilantro, lime juice, and a touch of jalapeño for a refreshing accompaniment to grilled fish or tacos.

2. **Light Summer Salads:** Incorporate white onions into light summer salads, where their gentle flavor won't overpower the delicate notes of fresh greens, fruits, and vinaigrette. The result is a crisp and refreshing salad that highlights the best of the season.

Sweet Onions: Nature's Candy in Every Bite

1. **Grilled Sweet Onion Rings:** Celebrate the natural sweetness of Vidalia or Walla Walla sweet onions by grilling thick slices. These caramelized onion rings make a delectable side dish, offering a balance of smokiness and sweetness that pairs well with grilled meats.

2. **Sweet Onion Jams:** Craft sweet onion jams to elevate your cheese platters or spread on sandwiches.

Simmer sweet onions with balsamic vinegar, honey, and a hint of thyme to create a versatile condiment that adds depth to both sweet and savory dishes.

Shallots: Subtle Sophistication in Culinary Creations

1. **Vinaigrettes and Dressings:** Shallots, with their mild yet sophisticated flavor, shine in homemade vinaigrettes and dressings. Combine finely minced shallots with olive oil, balsamic vinegar, and Dijon mustard for an elegant dressing that enhances the simplest salads.

2. **Creamy Sauces and Dips:** Incorporate shallots into creamy sauces and dips, where their subtle oniony notes complement rich and velvety textures. Whether blended into a classic béarnaise sauce or stirred into a sour cream-based dip, shallots add a touch of refinement.

Green Onions (Scallions): Freshness in Every Bite

1. **Garnishes for Soups and Noodles:** Green onions, with their mild and fresh flavor, make excellent garnishes for soups and noodle dishes. Finely chop

them and sprinkle on top of a bowl of miso soup or a plate of stir-fried noodles for a burst of color and freshness.

2. **Asian-inspired Stir-Fries:** Incorporate green onions into Asian-inspired stir-fries, where their crisp texture and mild onion flavor enhance the overall dish. Add them towards the end of cooking to preserve their vibrant green color and freshness.

Leeks: A Delicate Touch to Savory Creations

1. **Quiches and Frittatas:** Slice leeks into thin rounds and sauté them to add a delicate onion flavor to quiches and frittatas. Their mildness complements the richness of eggs and cheese, creating a harmonious balance of flavors.

2. **Creamy Potato Leek Soup:** Craft a classic creamy potato leek soup, where the subtle sweetness of leeks combines with the earthiness of potatoes. This comforting soup is a testament to the gentle elegance that leeks bring to savory creations.

Culinary Alchemy: Balancing Flavors for Wellness

1. Creating Flavorful Broths:

Use onion varieties, especially yellow onions, to create flavorful broths as a base for soups, stews, and sauces. The aromatic compounds released during the cooking process contribute to both the taste and potential health benefits of the final dish.

2. Balancing Sweet and Savory:

Experiment with the sweet and savory notes of onions in your dishes. Pair caramelized onions with savory meats, or add sweet onions to salads to strike a balance that pleases the palate and promotes a sense of culinary satisfaction.

Medicinal Elixirs: Herbal Infusions and Tonics

1. Onion-Infused Honey:

Craft onion-infused honey by combining finely chopped onions with raw honey. Allow the mixture to infuse for several days before straining. The resulting honey can be drizzled over warm tea or used as a sweet and savory glaze for roasted vegetables.

2. Onion Tonics for Immunity:

Prepare onion tonics by infusing sliced onions in apple cider vinegar. This potent elixir can be diluted with water and honey for a refreshing drink with potential immune-boosting benefits. Sip on this tonic during seasonal changes or when in need of a wellness pick-me-up.

Culinary Wisdom: The Healing Table

In the healing kitchen, the act of incorporating onions into daily meals transcends mere sustenance; it becomes a form of culinary wisdom. The flavors, aromas, and textures of onions contribute not only to the pleasure of eating but also to the holistic well-being of those gathered around the table.

Conclusion: A Symphony of Flavor and Wellness

As we embrace the art of incorporating onions into daily meals, let each chop, sauté, and simmer be a celebration of the healing potential found in nature's bounty. From the robustness of yellow onions to the elegance of shallots and the freshness of green onions, each variety brings its unique contribution to the culinary symphony.

In the chapters ahead, we will further explore the alchemy of crafting healing meals, combining the wisdom of herbal medicine with the joys of the kitchen. Let the healing table be a place where flavor and wellness harmonize, creating a symphony of delight for both body and soul.

Chapter 7

Onion Poultices and Compresses Harnessing Nature's Healing Power

In the realm of herbal medicine, onions emerge as unsung heroes, offering not only culinary delights but also a myriad of therapeutic applications. Among these, onion poultices and compresses stand out as time-honored remedies, harnessing the healing power of Alliums in a direct and targeted manner. In this chapter, we will delve into the art and science of creating onion poultices and compresses, exploring their applications, benefits, and the age-old wisdom that underlies their efficacy.

The Essence of Onion Poultices

Unveiling the Healing Potential

An onion poultice is a simple yet potent herbal preparation that involves applying crushed or heated onions directly to the skin. The natural compounds found in onions, such as allicin, flavonoids, and sulfur compounds, lend themselves to various therapeutic applications when used in this form.

Anti-Inflammatory Action

Onion poultices are renowned for their anti-inflammatory properties. When applied to the skin, the compounds in onions may help reduce inflammation, making poultices valuable for addressing conditions such as arthritis, joint pain, or localized swelling.

Drawing Out Toxins

The heat generated by an onion poultice can promote vasodilation, enhancing blood flow to the affected area. This increased circulation may aid in drawing out toxins and promoting the removal of waste products from the tissues, contributing to a detoxifying effect.

Crafting an Onion Poultice

Simple Steps for Effective Application

Ingredients:
- Fresh onions (preferably organic)
- Clean cloth or gauze
- Bandage or wrap

Steps:

1. **Choose Your Onions:** Select fresh onions based on the intended application. For anti-inflammatory purposes, red onions are often preferred, while white or yellow onions may be suitable for drawing out toxins.

2. **Peel and Crush:** Peel and crush the onions to release their juices. Use a mortar and pestle, grater, or blender to create a pulpy consistency. The goal is to extract the onion's natural compounds for maximum effectiveness.

3. **Prepare the Poultice:** Spread the crushed onions evenly on a clean cloth or gauze. Ensure that the poultice is large enough to cover the affected area adequately. The thickness of the poultice will depend on the desired intensity of the application.

4. **Application:** Place the onion poultice directly onto the affected area. Secure it in place with a bandage or wrap to ensure it remains in contact with the skin. Leave the poultice on for a duration appropriate to the specific condition (typically 15-30 minutes).

5. **Remove and Cleanse:** After the designated time, carefully remove the poultice. Cleanse the skin with warm water to remove any onion residue, and pat the area dry.

6. **Optional Heat Application:** For enhanced therapeutic effects, consider applying warmth to the poultice. This can be achieved by warming the crushed onions slightly before applying or by placing a warm compress over the poultice.

Targeted Applications: Tailoring Poultices to Needs

1. Arthritis and Joint Pain:

Onion poultices can be beneficial for individuals dealing with arthritis or joint pain. The anti-inflammatory properties of onions may help alleviate discomfort when applied directly to the affected area. Consider incorporating other anti-inflammatory herbs such as turmeric for added potency.

2. Muscle Strains and Sprains:

Apply an onion poultice to strained or sprained muscles to encourage blood flow, reduce inflammation, and potentially speed up the healing process. Combine with herbs like comfrey or arnica for added support in addressing muscle injuries.

3. Localized Swelling:

When dealing with localized swelling, such as insect bites or bruises, a cooling onion poultice can be soothing. Choose onions with anti-inflammatory properties and apply the poultice for a targeted, natural remedy.

The Art of Onion Compresses

Beyond Direct Application

Onion compresses extend the healing potential of onions to a broader range of applications. Compresses involve infusing water with the medicinal properties of onions, creating a solution that can be applied topically or used in other therapeutic ways.

Creating Onion Infusions

Ingredients:
- Fresh onions
- Hot water

- Clean cloth or towel
- Bandage or wrap

Steps:

1. **Peel and Slice the Onions:** Peel and slice fresh onions into thin rounds. The increased surface area enhances the extraction of medicinal compounds.

2. **Boil Water:** Bring water to a boil and then allow it to cool slightly. Pour the hot water over the sliced onions, creating an infusion. Allow the mixture to steep for 15-20 minutes.

3. **Strain and Cool:** Strain the onion-infused water to remove the onion pieces. Allow the solution to cool to a comfortable temperature for application.

4. **Application:** Soak a clean cloth or towel in the onion-infused water. Wring out excess liquid and apply the compress directly to the affected area. Secure with a bandage or wrap.

5. **Duration:** Leave the onion compress in place for 15-30 minutes, allowing the medicinal properties to be absorbed through the skin.

Multi-Purpose Uses

1. **Sunburn Relief:** Onion compresses can offer relief for sunburned skin. The anti-inflammatory properties of onions, coupled with the cooling effect of the compress, may alleviate pain and reduce redness.

2. **Congestion and Respiratory Support:** Inhaling the steam from onion compresses may provide respiratory benefits. Create an onion-infused water solution, allow it to cool slightly, and inhale the steam to potentially ease congestion or soothe respiratory discomfort.

Safety Considerations

Nurturing Wellness with Caution

While onion poultices and compresses can be powerful allies in promoting wellness, it's crucial to exercise caution and consider individual sensitivities.

Patch Test:

Before widespread application, conduct a patch test by applying a small amount of the onion poultice or compress to a small area of skin. Monitor for any adverse reactions, such as redness or irritation.

Eye Contact:

Take care to avoid contact with the eyes when applying onion poultices or compresses. If accidental contact occurs, rinse the eyes thoroughly with cool water.

Sensitivity and Allergies:

Individuals with sensitivities or allergies to onions should refrain from using onion poultices or compresses. Consider consulting with a healthcare professional for alternative remedies.

Conclusion: The Wisdom of Herbal Applications

In the age-old practice of herbal medicine, the simplicity and efficacy of onion poultices and compresses stand as a testament to the wisdom of harnessing nature's healing power. From reducing inflammation and drawing out toxins to providing relief for sunburn and respiratory discomfort, these applications offer a gentle and holistic approach to wellness.

As you explore the art of onion poultices and compresses, may you find not only relief for specific ailments but also a deeper connection to the timeless wisdom embedded in the natural world. In the upcoming chapters, we will continue our journey into the multifaceted realm of onion herbal medicine, unlocking more secrets and applications for the benefit of body, mind, and spirit

Chapter 8:

Onion Infusions and Teas Sipping Nature's Elixir: A Warm Embrace of Wellness

In the world of herbal medicine, the onion takes center stage not only in the culinary realm but also as a therapeutic elixir. The art of crafting onion infusions and teas unlocks the potential of these humble bulbs in a liquid form, providing a soothing and holistic approach to well-being. In this chapter, we will explore the nuanced practice of creating onion infusions and teas, delving into their diverse applications, benefits, and the comforting ritual of sipping nature's elixir.

Essence of Onion Infusions

Brewing Wellness in a Cup

An onion infusion is a concentrated liquid preparation achieved by steeping fresh onions in hot water. This gentle extraction process allows the water-soluble compounds present in onions, such as quercetin, flavonoids, and sulfur compounds, to infuse into the liquid, creating a potent beverage with potential health benefits.

Anti-Inflammatory Support:

The anti-inflammatory properties of onions, particularly quercetin, make onion infusions a soothing choice for individuals dealing with inflammatory conditions. Consuming these infusions may contribute to overall wellness by addressing inflammation at the cellular level.

Respiratory Comfort:

The aromatic compounds released during the infusion process can provide respiratory benefits. Inhaling the steam from a warm onion infusion may help ease congestion, soothe irritated airways, and promote a sense of respiratory comfort.

Crafting an Onion Infusion

Simple Steps for a Nourishing Brew

Ingredients:
- Fresh onions (preferably organic)
- Hot water

- Honey or lemon (optional, for flavor)

Steps:

1. **Choose Your Onions:** Select fresh onions based on the intended application. Red onions, with their rich quercetin content, are often preferred for their potential anti-inflammatory benefits.

2. **Peel and Slice:** Peel and slice the onions into thin rounds or small pieces. The increased surface area enhances the extraction of medicinal compounds.

3. **Boil Water:** Bring water to a boil and then allow it to cool slightly. Pour the hot water over the sliced onions, creating an infusion. Allow the mixture to steep for 10-15 minutes.

4. **Strain and Enjoy:** Strain the onion-infused water to remove the onion pieces. The resulting infusion can be consumed as is or enhanced with a touch of honey or lemon for flavor. Enjoy the infusion while it's warm.

Variations for Wellness

Tailoring Infusions to Individual Needs

1. **Anti-Inflammatory Blend:**

Combine red onions with anti-inflammatory herbs such as ginger and turmeric to create a potent infusion. This blend may offer enhanced support for individuals dealing with inflammatory conditions.

2. **Digestive Comfort:**

Infuse yellow onions with soothing herbs like peppermint or fennel to create a beverage that supports digestive health. Sip on this infusion after meals to aid digestion and reduce bloating.

3. **Immune-Boosting Elixir:**

Enhance the immune-boosting potential of onion infusions by incorporating immune-supportive herbs like echinacea or elderberry. This warming elixir can be particularly comforting during cold and flu seasons.

Onion Teas: A Culinary Symphony for the Palate

Savoring Nature's Symphony in a Teacup

Onion teas elevate the experience of consuming onions for wellness by combining the therapeutic properties of onions with a delightful array of complementary herbs and spices. These teas not only offer potential health benefits but also bring a symphony of flavors to the palate.

Balancing Sweet and Savory:

Onion teas often incorporate sweet and savory elements to create a harmonious balance of flavors. The sweetness of honey or the warmth of spices like cinnamon can complement the pungency of onions, making the tea not only beneficial but also enjoyable.

Culinary Alchemy:

Infusing onion teas with herbs like thyme, rosemary, or basil adds layers of complexity to the flavor profile. This culinary alchemy transforms a simple tea into a sensory experience, engaging both taste and aroma.

Crafting an Onion Tea

Aromatic Blends for Pleasure and Wellness

Ingredients:
- Fresh onions (preferably organic)
- Hot water
- Additional herbs and spices (e.g., ginger, cinnamon, thyme)

• Honey or lemon (optional, for flavor)

Steps:

1. **Choose Your Onions and Additional Ingredients:** Select fresh onions and any additional herbs or spices based on the desired flavor profile and potential health benefits.

2. **Peel and Slice:** Peel and slice the onions into thin rounds or small pieces. If using other herbs or spices, prepare them accordingly.

3. **Boil Water:** Bring water to a boil and then allow it to cool slightly. Pour the hot water over the sliced onions and any additional ingredients, creating a flavorful tea base. Allow the mixture to steep for 10-15 minutes.

4. **Strain and Enjoy:** Strain the tea to remove the onion pieces and any other solid components. The resulting tea can be consumed as is or enhanced with honey or lemon for flavor. Sip on the tea while it's warm.

Culinary Creativity: Blending Flavors for Pleasure

1. Herbal Symphony:

Blend onions with aromatic herbs like thyme, rosemary, and sage for a savory tea that engages the senses. This herbal symphony not only offers potential health benefits but also provides a delightful and comforting experience.

2. Spiced Elixirs:

Explore the world of spiced onion teas by incorporating warming spices like ginger, cinnamon, and cardamom. This spiced elixir can be particularly comforting during colder months, providing a sense of warmth and well-being.

Safety Considerations

Nurturing Wellness with Caution

While onion infusions and teas offer a gentle and natural approach to wellness, it's important to consider individual sensitivities and exercise caution.

Moderation:

Consume onion infusions and teas in moderation. Excessive intake may lead to stomach discomfort or digestive issues, particularly in individuals with sensitive stomachs.

Allergies:

Individuals with allergies to onions or related vegetables should avoid onion infusions and teas. Consider consulting with a healthcare professional for alternative remedies.

Individual Tolerance:

Pay attention to individual tolerance levels. If experiencing any adverse reactions, such as gastrointestinal discomfort or skin irritation, discontinue use and seek guidance from a healthcare professional.

Conclusion: A Sip of Nature's Comfort

In the gentle infusion of onions into elixirs and teas, we discover a soothing and comforting ritual that transcends the mere act of consumption. Sipping on nature's comfort through these warm brews not only offers potential health benefits but also allows us to partake in the timeless wisdom embedded in the natural world.

As you embrace the art of crafting onion infusions and teas, may each sip be a moment of connection with the healing essence of nature. In the forthcoming chapters, we will continue our exploration of the multifaceted world of onion herbal medicine, unveiling more secrets and applications for the benefit of body, mind, and spirit.

Chapter 9

Onions in Traditional Medicine Practices Tapping into Centuries of Wisdom

As we delve deeper into the world of herbal medicine, the onion emerges as a venerable ally, celebrated not only in kitchens around the globe but also within the annals of traditional medicine practices. For centuries, cultures worldwide have recognized and harnessed the healing potential of onions, weaving them into diverse therapeutic traditions. In this chapter, we will embark on a journey through time and traditions, exploring the rich tapestry of how onions have been revered and utilized in traditional medicine practices across different cultures.

Ancient Roots of Healing

A Symbol of Life and Vitality

In ancient civilizations, the onion was revered not only for its culinary virtues but also for its symbolic significance. Egyptians, Greeks, and Romans considered onions as a symbol of life and vitality. The layered structure of the onion, reminiscent of the cycles of life and regeneration, captured the imaginations of these ancient cultures.

Egyptian Elixirs:

In ancient Egypt, onions were not only consumed as a dietary staple but also utilized in medicinal elixirs. The pungent bulbs were believed to have protective qualities, with the ability to ward off various ailments.

Greek and Roman Remedies:

Hippocrates, the ancient Greek physician known as the "Father of Medicine," prescribed onions for various health conditions. Romans, too, valued onions for their medicinal properties and employed them in poultices, tonics, and topical applications.

Ayurveda: The Ancient Healing System of India

Balancing Energies for Holistic Wellness

In the ancient Indian healing system of Ayurveda, onions find a place among the vast array of herbs and foods used to balance the three doshas—Vata, Pitta, and Kapha. Ayurvedic practitioners recognize the warming and stimulating qualities of onions, which can be beneficial for pacifying certain imbalances.

Vata Pacifying:

Onions, with their pungent and heating attributes, are considered Vata-pacifying in Ayurveda. Vata, associated with the elements of air and space, can benefit from the grounding and warming nature of onions.

Digestive Aid:

Ayurveda acknowledges the digestive prowess of onions. Incorporating them into meals is believed to stimulate agni, the digestive fire, and enhance the assimilation of nutrients.

Traditional Chinese Medicine: Balancing Yin and Yang

Harmonizing Energies for Optimal Health

In Traditional Chinese Medicine (TCM), the principles of Yin and Yang guide the understanding of balance within the body. Onions, classified as pungent and warming, are considered to have properties that can harmonize these energies when used appropriately.

Warming Nature:

Onions are regarded as energetically warm in TCM. This warmth is believed to support the Yang aspect of the body, promoting circulation and dispelling cold.

Dispelling Dampness:

TCM views onions as having the ability to dispel dampness within the body. Dampness is associated with stagnation and imbalance, and onions are employed to foster a more harmonious internal environment.

Folk Medicine Traditions: Europe and Beyond

Healing Wisdom Passed Through Generations

In European folk medicine, onions were prized for their accessibility and versatility. Commonly found in kitchen gardens, onions became staples in home remedies passed down through generations.

Culinary and Medicinal Synergy:

Folk medicine traditions often blurred the lines between culinary and medicinal applications. Onion soups, tonics, and poultices were crafted to address a range of ailments, from respiratory issues to joint pain.

Warding off Illness:

Folklore in various European cultures suggested hanging strings of onions in homes during the cold and flu season to ward off illness. The pungent aroma was believed to purify the air and protect against infectious agents.

Native American Herbal Wisdom

Harnessing Nature's Bounty for Healing

Native American tribes embraced the bounty of the land, using indigenous plants, including wild onions, for medicinal purposes. The Cherokee, for example, utilized wild onions as part of their healing practices.

Respiratory Support:

Native Americans recognized the respiratory benefits of wild onions. Infusions and poultices made from these plants were employed to address coughs, colds, and respiratory congestion.

Ceremonial Significance:

Beyond their medicinal uses, onions held ceremonial significance in some Native American cultures. The symbolism of renewal and life associated with the layers of the onion mirrored their spiritual beliefs.

Unveiling Onions in Islamic Medicine

Ancient Wisdom Rooted in Faith

In Islamic medicine, onions are celebrated for their potential health benefits, and references to their healing properties can be found in ancient texts. Islamic scholars, including Ibn Sina (Avicenna), recognized the therapeutic virtues of onions.

Antibacterial Properties:

Islamic medicine acknowledges the antibacterial properties of onions. Consuming onions was believed to contribute to the body's ability to resist infections and maintain overall health.

Culinary and Medicinal Fusion:

Onions seamlessly blended into the culinary and medicinal traditions of Islamic cultures. From flavoring dishes to preparing tonics, the multifaceted use of onions showcased their esteemed status.

African Traditional Medicine: A Tapestry of Diversity

Cultural Richness in Healing Practices

Across the diverse landscapes of Africa, traditional medicine practices vary, each reflecting the unique cultural tapestry of the region. Onions, readily available in many parts of Africa, have found a place in diverse healing rituals.

Gastrointestinal Harmony:

Traditional healers in some African cultures have employed onions for addressing gastrointestinal issues. Infusions, teas, or poultices made from onions may be used to soothe digestive discomfort.

Rituals and Symbolism:

Onions may hold symbolic significance in certain African healing rituals. Their use extends beyond the physical realm, often involving spiritual and symbolic dimensions within the cultural context.

Onions in Contemporary Herbalism

Bridging Tradition and Modern Practices

As we navigate the complex landscape of modern herbalism, the wisdom of traditional medicine practices continues to shape the use of onions for health and well-being. Herbalists draw upon both ancient knowledge and contemporary research to incorporate onions into holistic healing approaches.

Anti-Inflammatory Applications:

The anti-inflammatory properties of onions, particularly attributed to compounds like quercetin, continue to be recognized in contemporary herbalism. Onion extracts or infusions may be recommended for addressing inflammation-related conditions.

Cardiometabolic Support:

Research exploring the potential cardiovascular benefits of onions, including their impact on cholesterol levels and blood pressure, aligns with both traditional and modern perspectives on the holistic well-being promoted by these bulbs.

Safety Considerations and Precautions

Guiding Principles for Responsible Use

While onions have a long history of safe use in traditional medicine practices, it's important to approach their application with consideration for individual sensitivities and variations in health conditions.

Individual Allergies:

Individuals with known allergies to onions or related vegetables should exercise caution. In cases of allergic reactions, ranging from mild skin irritation to more severe symptoms, it's advisable to avoid onion-based remedies.

Digestive Sensitivities:

Some individuals may experience digestive discomfort, bloating, or heartburn when consuming onions. Monitoring individual responses and adjusting the dosage or form of administration can help mitigate potential issues.

Consulting Healthcare Professionals:

Those with underlying health conditions, pregnant individuals, or individuals taking specific medications should consult with healthcare professionals before incorporating onion-based remedies into their wellness routines.

Conclusion: A Tapestry of Healing Traditions

In exploring the role of onions in traditional medicine practices, we traverse continents and centuries, witnessing the universal reverence for these humble bulbs in diverse cultural landscapes. Whether steeped in the wisdom of Ayurveda, integrated into the harmonizing principles of Traditional Chinese Medicine, or woven into the rich tapestry of African healing rituals, onions persist as symbols of life, vitality, and holistic well-being.

As we bridge the wisdom of ancient traditions with modern perspectives, may the exploration of onions in traditional medicine practices inspire a deeper appreciation for the interconnectedness of humanity and nature. In the chapters ahead, we will continue our journey into the multifaceted realm of onion herbal medicine, unveiling more secrets and applications for the benefit of body, mind, and spirit.

Chapter 10:

Onion Supplements and Future Trends Unveiling the Potential: From Kitchen Staple to Nutraceutical

As the landscape of health and wellness evolves, the humble onion, long celebrated in culinary traditions and herbal medicine, takes on new significance as a potential nutraceutical. The emergence of onion supplements marks a departure from traditional applications, opening doors to innovative ways of harnessing the therapeutic properties of Alliums. In this chapter, we will explore the realm of onion supplements, their benefits, and the evolving trends that may shape the future of onion-based nutraceuticals.

The Rise of Nutraceuticals

A Fusion of Nutrition and Pharmaceuticals

Nutraceuticals represent a fusion of nutrition and pharmaceuticals, encapsulating the idea that certain foods or food components may provide health benefits beyond basic nutrition. Onions, rich in bioactive compounds, are poised to make a significant contribution to this growing sector.

Bioactive Compounds:

The therapeutic potential of onions lies in their bioactive compounds, including quercetin, sulfur compounds, and flavonoids. These compounds have been associated with antioxidant, anti-inflammatory, and other health-promoting effects.

Scientific Exploration:

Research into the medicinal properties of onions has fueled interest in developing nutraceutical products that harness the concentrated benefits of these bioactive compounds. Onion supplements offer a convenient and standardized way to deliver these compounds in specific doses.

The Potential Benefits of Onion Supplements

Targeted Support for Well-Being

Onion supplements hold the promise of delivering concentrated doses of bioactive compounds, offering targeted support for various aspects of health and well-being.

Cardiometabolic Health:

Studies suggest that onion-derived compounds may contribute to cardiometabolic health by positively influencing factors such as cholesterol levels, blood pressure, and glucose metabolism. Onion supplements could be designed to specifically address these aspects.

Anti-Inflammatory Effects:

The anti-inflammatory properties of quercetin, a prominent compound in onions, have implications for conditions associated with inflammation. Onion supplements may offer a standardized source of quercetin for individuals seeking natural anti-inflammatory support.

Antioxidant Defense:

Onions are rich in antioxidants that help neutralize free radicals in the body. Supplemental forms could enhance antioxidant defense, potentially supporting overall cellular health and reducing oxidative stress.

Immune Modulation:

The immune-modulating effects of onion compounds may contribute to immune system balance. Onion supplements could be explored for their potential to support immune function and resilience.

Innovations in Supplement Formulations

Beyond Traditional Capsules

As onion supplements gain popularity, innovation in formulation methods and delivery systems is shaping the landscape. Beyond traditional capsules, various forms of onion supplements are emerging to cater to diverse preferences and absorption profiles.

Powders and Extracts:

Onion supplements are available in powdered forms and concentrated extracts. These formulations may provide higher concentrations of bioactive compounds, allowing for lower dosage and potentially improved bioavailability.

Softgels and Gummies:

Softgel capsules and gummy formulations are becoming popular choices for those seeking alternative delivery methods. These formats offer convenience and may appeal to individuals who find traditional capsules less palatable.

Functional Foods and Beverages:

The integration of onion extracts into functional foods and beverages is an exciting trend. From energy bars to health drinks, incorporating onion-derived compounds into everyday consumables widens the scope of reaching diverse consumer preferences.

Future Trends in Onion Nutraceuticals

Exploring the Horizon

As the field of nutraceuticals continues to expand, several trends and developments may shape the future of onion-based supplements.

Personalized Nutrition:

Advancements in personalized nutrition may lead to the development of onion supplements tailored to individual health needs. Genetic profiling and biomarker analysis could guide formulations that address specific health concerns for each individual.

Combination Formulas:

Future onion supplements may feature combination formulas, blending onion-derived compounds with other botanicals, vitamins, or minerals for synergistic effects. These formulations could target multiple aspects of well-being in a single supplement.

Sustainable Sourcing and Processing:

With a growing emphasis on sustainability, future trends may prioritize ethically sourced onions and eco-friendly processing methods. This shift aligns with consumer preferences for products that consider environmental impact.

Bioavailability Enhancement:

Ongoing research may uncover ways to enhance the bioavailability of onion-derived compounds, ensuring optimal absorption and effectiveness. Innovations in delivery systems or co-formulation with absorption-enhancing agents could play a role in this advancement.

Clinical Validation:

As onion supplements gain traction, there may be an increased focus on rigorous clinical trials to validate their efficacy. Well-designed studies could provide scientific evidence supporting the use of onion supplements for specific health conditions.

Safety Considerations and Recommendations

Nurturing Health with Caution

While onion supplements hold promise, it's essential to approach their use with care, considering individual sensitivities and potential interactions with medications.

Allergies and Sensitivities:

Individuals with known allergies to onions or related vegetables should exercise caution when considering onion supplements. Allergic reactions, ranging from mild skin irritation to more severe symptoms, may occur.

Digestive Sensitivities:

Some individuals may experience digestive discomfort, bloating, or heartburn when consuming onion supplements. Adjusting the dosage or form of administration may help mitigate potential digestive issues.

Interactions with Medications:

Individuals taking specific medications, especially those with known interactions with onion compounds (e.g., blood thinners), should consult healthcare professionals before incorporating onion supplements into their routines.

Quality and Purity:

Choosing high-quality, standardized supplements from reputable manufacturers is crucial to ensure purity and potency. Consumers should look for products that undergo third-party testing for quality assurance.

Conclusion: Navigating the Future of Onion Nutraceuticals

In the ever-evolving landscape of health and wellness, onion supplements represent a promising frontier, offering concentrated doses of bioactive compounds for targeted support. As research and innovation continue to shape the field of nutraceuticals, onions, with their rich history in culinary and herbal traditions, contribute to the tapestry of natural approaches to well-being.

As we navigate the future of onion nutraceuticals, may the exploration of innovative formulations, personalized approaches, and sustainability considerations inspire a deeper appreciation for the potential of these humble bulbs to support health. In the upcoming chapters, we will continue our journey into the multifaceted realm of onion herbal medicine, uncovering more secrets and applications for the benefit of body, mind, and spirit.

www.ingramcontent.com/pod-product-compliance
Lightning Source LLC
Chambersburg PA
CBHW081204290526
45796CB00010B/333